AF596618

BEST FOOD FOR PREGNANCY

Healthy Diet For The Mother & Baby Well-being

Theresa Abraham

All rights reserved. No part of this publication may be reproduced, distributed, or transmitted in any form or by any means,including photocopying, recording, or other electronic or mechanical methods, without the prior written permission of the publisher, except in the case of brief quotations embodied in critical reviews and certain other noncommercial uses permitted by copyright law.

Copyright © Theresa Abraham, 2022

Table of contents

Chapter 1

PREGNANCY

Pregnancy happens when a sperm fertilizes an egg after it's released from the ovary during ovulation. The fertilized egg then travels down into the uterus, where implantation happens. A successful implantation results in pregnancy.

On average, a full-term pregnancy lasts 40 weeks. Several elements might affect a pregnancy. Women who obtain an early pregnancy diagnosis and prenatal care are more likely to enjoy a healthy pregnancy and give birth to a healthy baby.

Knowing what to anticipate throughout the complete pregnant term is vital for monitoring both your health and the health of the baby. If you'd prefer to avoid conception, there are additional effective kinds of birth control you should keep in mind.

Symptoms Of Pregnancy

You may notice certain signs and symptoms before you ever take a pregnancy test. Others may show weeks later, as your hormone levels alter.

Missed period

Missing menstruation is one of the early signs of pregnancy (and maybe the most typical one). However, a missing period doesn't always imply you're pregnant, particularly if your cycle tends to be erratic.

There are several health issues other than pregnancy that might cause late or missing menstruation.

Headache

Headaches are typical in early pregnancy. They're frequently caused by changing hormone levels and increased blood volume. Contact your doctor if your headaches don't go away or are very severe.

Spotting

Some women may have minor bleeding and spotting in early pregnancy. This bleeding is most typically the outcome of implantation. Implantation normally happens one to two weeks following conception.

Early pregnancy bleeding may also develop from very modest issues such as an infection or discomfort. The latter typically affects the surface of the cervix (which is especially sensitive during pregnancy).

Bleeding may also occasionally suggest a major pregnancy issue, such as miscarriage, ectopic pregnancy, or placenta previa. Always contact your doctor if you're worried.

Weight gain

You should anticipate gaining between 1 and 4 pounds in your first few months of pregnancy. Weight gain becomes more obvious at the beginning of your second trimester.

Pregnancy-induced hypertension

High blood pressure, or hypertension, sometimes occurs during pregnancy. A lot of variables may raise your risk, including:

being overweight or obese

smoking

having a history or a family history of pregnancy-induced hypertension

Heartburn

Hormones generated during pregnancy may occasionally loosen the valve between your stomach and esophagus. When stomach acid spills out, this might result in heartburn.

Constipation

Hormone changes during early pregnancy might slow down your digestive system. As a consequence, you may get constipated.

Cramps

As the muscles in your uterus begin to stretch and develop, you may experience a tugging feeling that mimics menstruation pains. If spotting or blood occurs with your cramps, it might signify a miscarriage or an ectopic pregnancy.

Back pain

Hormones and tension in the muscles are the primary causes of back discomfort in early pregnancy. Later on, your increased weight and shifting center of gravity may contribute to your back discomfort. Around half of all pregnant women feel back discomfort throughout their pregnancy.

Anemia

Pregnant women have an increased risk of anemia, which produces symptoms such as lightheadedness and dizziness.

The syndrome may lead to preterm delivery and low birth weight. Prenatal care frequently includes screening for anemia.

Depression

Between 14 and 23 percent of all pregnant women suffer depression throughout their pregnancy. The various bodily and mental changes you undergo might be significant reasons.

Be careful to notify your doctor if you don't feel like your regular self.

Insomnia

Insomnia is another typical symptom of early pregnancy. Stress, physical pain, and hormonal fluctuations all be contributory reasons. A balanced diet, excellent sleep habits, and yoga stretches may all help you obtain a good night's sleep.

Breast changes

Breast changes are one of the earliest apparent indications of pregnancy. Even before you're far enough along for a positive test, your breasts may begin to feel sensitive, swollen, and generally heavy or full. Your nipples may also get bigger and more sensitive, and the areolae may darken.

Acne

Because of elevated androgen hormones, many women have acne in early pregnancy. These hormones may make your face oilier, which can block pores. Pregnancy acne is generally transient and clears up once the baby is delivered.

Vomiting

Vomiting is a component of “morning sickness,” a frequent symptom that normally starts during the first four months. Morning sickness is frequently the first indicator that you’re pregnant. Increased hormones during early pregnancy are the major culprits.

Hip discomfort

Hip discomfort is prevalent throughout pregnancy and tends to intensify in late pregnancy. It may have several reasons, including:

the strain on your ligaments

sciatica changes in your posture

a heavier uterus

Diarrhea

Diarrhea and other stomach issues occur often during pregnancy. Hormone changes, a changing diet, and additional stress are all plausible factors. If diarrhea lasts longer than a few days, call your doctor to make sure you don't get dehydrated.

Stress And Pregnancy

While pregnancy is normally a pleasant time, it may sometimes be a source of stress. A new baby brings enormous changes to your body, your connections, and even your money. Don't hesitate to approach your doctor for support if you begin to feel overwhelmed.

Summary

If you suspect you may be pregnant, you shouldn't depend exclusively on these signs and symptoms for proof. Taking a home pregnancy test or contacting your doctor for lab testing may confirm a probable pregnancy.

Many of these signs and symptoms might also be caused by other health issues, such as premenstrual syndrome (PMS). Learn more about the early signs of pregnancy – such as how soon they'll occur if you miss your period.

Pregnancy Symptoms: 10 Early Signs That You May Be Pregnant

Pregnancy week by week
Pregnancy weeks are split into three trimesters, each one featuring medical milestones for both you and the baby.

First trimester
A baby develops fast throughout the first trimester (wccks 1 to 12). The fetus starts growing its brain, spinal cord, and organs. The baby's heart will also begin to beat.

During the first trimester, the likelihood of a miscarriage is rather high. According to the American College of Obstetricians and Gynecologists (ACOG), it's believed that roughly 1 in 10 pregnancies terminates in miscarriage and that about 85 percent of these occur in the first trimester.

Second trimester
During the second trimester of pregnancy (weeks 13 to 27), your healthcare practitioner will likely conduct an anatomy scan ultrasound.

This examination evaluates the fetus's body for any developmental problems. The test findings might also indicate the sex of your baby if you choose to find out before the baby is born.

You'll probably begin to feel your baby move, kick, and punch inside of your uterus.

After 23 weeks, a baby in utero is declared "viable." This suggests that it might survive life outside of your womb. Babies born this early sometimes have major medical concerns. Your baby has a far higher chance of being delivered healthy the longer you can carry the pregnancy.

Third trimester

During the third trimester (weeks 28 to 40), your weight increases may speed up, and you may feel more exhausted. Your infant can now perceive light as well as open and shut their eyes. Their bones are also produced.

As labor approaches, you may experience pelvic pain, and your feet may swell. Contractions that don't progress to labor, known as Braxton-Hicks contractions, may start to occur in the weeks before you deliver.

Summary

Every pregnancy is different, although developments will most likely occur within this broad time range. Find out more about the changes you and your baby will endure during the trimesters.

Pregnancy Testing

Home pregnancy tests are highly accurate after the first day of your missing menstruation. If you obtain a positive result on a home pregnancy test, you should arrange an appointment with your doctor straight away. An ultrasound will be performed to confirm and date your pregnancy.

Pregnancy is detected by detecting the body's levels of human chorionic gonadotropin (hCG). Also referred to as the pregnancy hormone, hCG is created following implantation. However, it may not be discovered until after you miss a period.

After you miss a period, hCG levels grow fast. hCG is identified using either a urine or a blood test.

Urine tests may be offered in a doctor's office, and they're the same as the ones you may perform at home.

Blood tests may be conducted in a laboratory. hCG blood tests are roughly as accurate as home pregnancy tests. The distinction is that blood tests may be conducted as soon as six days following ovulation.

The sooner you can confirm you're pregnant, the better. An early diagnosis will help you to take better care of your baby's health. Get additional information about pregnancy tests, such as recommendations for avoiding a "false negative" result.

Pregnancy And Vaginal Discharge

An increase in vaginal discharge is one of the early indicators of pregnancy. Your production of discharge may rise as early as one to two weeks after conception before you've even missed a period.

As your pregnancy advances, you'll continue to generate increased volumes of discharge. The discharge will also likely get heavier and occur more often. It's generally heaviest near the conclusion of your pregnancy.

During the final weeks of your pregnancy, your discharge may contain streaks of thick mucus and blood. This is nicknamed "the gory show." It may be an early symptom of labor. You should let your doctor know if you experience any bleeding.

Normal vaginal discharge, called leukorrhea, is thin and either clear or milky white. It's also mild-smelling.

If your discharge is yellow, green, or gray with a strong, unpleasant odor, it's deemed abnormal. The abnormal discharge might be an indication of an infection or a problem with your pregnancy, particularly if there's redness, itching, or vulvar swelling.

If you suspect you have abnormal vaginal discharge, let your healthcare practitioner know immediately. Learn more about vaginal discharge during pregnancy.

Pregnancy And Urinary Tract Infections (UTIs)

Urinary tract infections (UTIs) are one of the most frequent problems women suffer during pregnancy. Bacteria can get inside a woman's urethra, or urinary tract, and can move up into the bladder. The fetus exerts increased strain on the bladder, which might cause the germs to be trapped, producing an infection.

Symptoms of a UTI generally include discomfort and burning or frequent urination. You may also experience:
cloudy or blood-tinged urine
pelvic pain
lower back ache
fever, nausea, and vomiting
Nearly 18 percent of pregnant women have a UTI. You may help avoid these infections by emptying your bladder often, particularly before and after intercourse. Drink lots of water to keep hydrated. Avoid using douches and strong soaps in the genital region.

Contact your healthcare practitioner if you develop symptoms of a UTI. Infections during pregnancy may be harmful because they raise the risk of early labor.
When identified early, most UTIs may be treated with medications that are efficient against bacteria but remain safe for use during pregnancy.

Pregnancy or PMS

The symptoms of early pregnancy might sometimes mirror those of premenstrual syndrome (PMS). It may be tough for a woman to determine whether she's pregnant or merely experiencing the start of another menstrual cycle.

A woman must know as soon as possible whether she's pregnant so that she can obtain good prenatal care. She may also wish to adopt specific lifestyle adjustments, such as refraining from drinking, taking prenatal vitamins, and improving her nutrition.

Taking a pregnancy test is the best, and simplest, the method to establish whether it's PMS or early pregnancy. You may take a home test or see your healthcare physician.

Some common symptoms of both PMS and early pregnancy include:

breast pain

bleeding

mood shifts

fatigue

food sensitivities

cramping

Underlying Conditions

Underlying health issues such as high blood pressure, diabetes, or cardiovascular disease will raise your risk of pregnancy difficulties. Other instances include:

cancer

renal disease

epilepsy

If you have one of these conditions, ensure that it's appropriately monitored and treated during your pregnancy. Otherwise, it may lead to miscarriage, poor fetal development, and birth abnormalities.

Other Risk Factors

Other conditions that might influence an otherwise healthy pregnancy include:

multiple-birth pregnancies, such as twins or triplets

Infections, including STDs

being overweight or obese

Anemia

Pregnancy complications

Pregnancy difficulties might include the baby's health, the mother's health, or both. They may arise during pregnancy or delivery.

Common pregnancy concerns include:

high blood pressure

gestational diabetes
preeclampsia
preterm labor
miscarriage
Addressing them early may reduce the effects done to the mother or the infant. Know your alternatives when it comes to addressing pregnancy issues.

Pregnancy And Labor
Sometime after your fourth month of pregnancy, you may begin to feel Braxton-Hick contractions or false labor. They're perfectly natural and help to prepare your uterus for the work ahead of genuine labor.

Braxton-Hick contractions don't occur at regular intervals, and they don't rise in strength. If you feel consistent contractions before week 37, it might be premature labor. If this happens, contact your healthcare practitioner for aid.

Early labor
Labor contractions are commonly classed as early labor contractions and active labor contractions. Early labor contractions last between 30 and 45 seconds. They may be far apart at first, but towards

the end of early labor, contractions will be around five minutes apart.

Your water can break early during labor, or your doctor may break it for you later on during your labor. When the cervix starts to open, you'll observe a blood-tinged discharge covering the mucus plug.

Active labor

In active labor, the cervix dilates, and the contractions become closer together and become more severe.

If you're in active labor, you should phone your healthcare practitioner and proceed to your birth location. If you're unclear if it's active labor, it's still a good idea to phone and check-in.

Labor pain

Pain will be at its height during active labor. Have a talk with your doctor about your preferred approach to coping with pain.

You may pick drug-free methods such as meditation, yoga, or listening to music.

If you want to treat your pain with medications, your doctor will need to know whether to use analgesics or anesthetics.

Analgesics, such as meperidine (Demerol), lessen the pain yet enable you to maintain some sensation. Anesthetics, such as an epidural, inhibit some muscle action and fully suppress the pain.

Summary

Whether you're planning for a vaginal or cesarean birth, you may feel worried as your due date approaches. Know what to anticipate with this guide to the various phases of labor.

Prognosis

You're likely to pass through each week of your pregnancy without too much problem. Pregnancy comes with numerous changes to your body, but those changes don't necessarily have a major influence on your health.

However, some lifestyle choices may either support or actively hurt your baby's growth.

Some actions that can keep you and your baby healthy include:

taking a multivitamin
getting sufficient sleep
practicing safe sex
receiving a flu shot
visiting your doctor

Some things you'll want to avoid include:
smoking
drinking alcohol
consuming raw meat, deli meat, or unpasteurized dairy products
sitting in a hot tub or sauna
gaining too much weight

Medications

It might be challenging to identify which drugs you can use during pregnancy and which ones you should avoid. You'll have to evaluate the advantages to your health against any hazards to the growing baby.

Ask your healthcare practitioner about any medications you may use, including OTC ones for mild conditions such as headaches.

Learning or relearning all the regulations of pregnancy may be difficult, particularly if you're having your first kid. Feel better prepared with this handy list of pregnant do's and don'ts.

Chapter 2

HEALTHY DIET

A good diet helps to guard against malnutrition in all its manifestations, as well as noncommunicable illnesses such as diabetes, heart disease, stroke, and cancer.

Unhealthy food and lack of physical exercise are primary worldwide dangers to health.

Healthy eating habits start early in life - breastfeeding supports healthy growth and enhances cognitive development, and may have longer-term health advantages such as lowering the risk of being overweight or obese and having NCDs later in life.

Energy intake (calories) should be in harmony with energy expenditure. To prevent harmful weight gain, total fat should not exceed 30% of total calorie consumption. Intake of saturated fats should be less than 10% of total calorie intake, and intake of trans-fats less than 1% of total energy intake, with a shift in fat consumption away from saturated fats and trans-fats to unsaturated fats, and towards the objective of eliminating industrially-produced trans-fats.

Limiting consumption of free sugars to less than 10% of total energy intake is part of a healthy diet. A further decrease to less than 5% of total calorie consumption is proposed for further health advantages.
Keeping salt consumption to less than 5 g per day (equal to sodium intake of less than 2 g per day) helps to avoid hypertension, and minimizes the risk of heart disease and stroke in the adult population.

Consuming a balanced diet throughout the life course helps to avoid malnutrition in all its manifestations as well as a spectrum of noncommunicable illnesses (NCDs) and disorders. However, increasing manufacturing of processed foods, rapid urbanization, and changing lifestyles have contributed to a change in dietary trends. Individuals are increasingly eating more meals heavy in calories, fats, free sugars, and salt sodium, and many people do not consume enough fruit, vegetables, and other dietary fiber such as whole grains.

The specific make-up of a diverse, balanced, and nutritious diet will vary based on individual factors (e.g. age, gender, lifestyle, and degree of physical activity), cultural background, regionally accessible foods, and dietary habits. However, the core concepts of what defines a healthy diet remain the same.

For Adults

A healthy diet contains the following:

Fruit, vegetables, legumes (e.g. lentils and beans), nuts, and whole grains (e.g. unprocessed maize, millet, oats, wheat, and brown rice).

At least 400 g (i.e. five servings) of fruit and vegetables each day, avoiding potatoes, sweet potatoes, cassava, and other starchy roots.

Less than 10% of total energy intake from free sugars, which is comparable to 50 g (or approximately 12 level teaspoons) for a person of healthy body weight eating roughly 2000 calories per day, but preferably is less than 5% of total energy intake for extra health advantages. Free sugars are any sugars added to foods or beverages by the manufacturer, chef, or consumer, as well as sugars naturally found in honey, syrups, fruit juices, and fruit juice concentrates.

Less than 30% of total calorie consumption comes from fats. Unsaturated fats (found in fish, avocado, and nuts, and in sunflower, soybean, canola, and olive oils) are preferable to saturated fats (found in fatty meat, butter, palm, and coconut oil, cream, cheese, ghee, and lard) and trans-fats of all kinds, including both industrially-produced trans-fats (found in baked and fried foods, and pre-packaged snacks and foods, such as frozen pizza, pies, cookies, biscuits, wafers, and cooking oils and spreads) and ruminant trans-fats (found in meat and dairy foods from ruminant animals, such as cows, sheep, goats, and camels) (found in meat and dairy foods from ruminant animals, such as cows, sheep, goats, and camels). It is proposed that the consumption of saturated fats be decreased to less than 10% of total energy intake and trans fats to less than 1% of total energy intake. In particular, industrially-produced trans-fats are not part of a healthy diet and should be avoided.

Less than 5g of salt (equal to around one teaspoon) each day. Salt should be iodized.

For Infants And Young Children

In the first 2 years of a child's life, ideal food stimulates healthy growth and enhances cognitive development. It also lowers the probability of becoming overweight or obese and having NCDs later in life.
Advice on a healthy diet for babies and children is similar to that for adults, however, the following things are particularly important:

Infants should be breastfed exclusively during the first 6 months of life.

Infants should be breastfed continuously until 2 years of age and beyond.

From 6 months of age, breast milk should be reinforced with a variety of acceptable, safe, and nutrient-dense foods.

Salt and sugar should not be added to complimenting meals.

Practical Advice On Maintaining A Healthy Diets.
Fruit and vegetables

Eating at least 400 g, or five servings, of fruit and vegetables per day lessens the risk of NCDs and helps to reach an optimal daily intake of dietary fiber.

Fruit and vegetable intake may be boosted by:
always incorporating vegetables in meals
eating fresh fruit and raw vegetables as snacks; eating fresh fruit and vegetables that are in season and seating a range of fruit and vegetables.

Fats

Reducing the amount of total fat consumption to less than 30% of total calorie intake helps to prevent hazardous weight gain in the adult population. Also, the risk of developing NCDs is lowered by:
reducing saturated fats to less than 10% of total energy consumption; reducing trans-fats to less than 1% of total energy intake; and replacing both saturated fats and trans-fats with unsaturated fats – in particular, with polyunsaturated fats.

Fat intake, especially saturated fat and industrially-produced trans-fat intake, can be reduced by:
steaming or boiling instead of frying when cooking

replacing butter, lard, and ghee with oils rich in polyunsaturated fats, such as soybean, canola (rapeseed), corn, safflower, and sunflower oils

eating reduced-fat dairy foods and lean meats, or trimming visible fat from meat; and limiting the consumption of baked and fried foods, and pre-packaged snacks and foods (e.g. doughnuts, cakes, pies, cookies, biscuits, and wafers) that contain industrially-produced trans-fats.

Salt, sodium, and potassium

Most adults consume too much sodium through salt (equal to swallowing an average of 9–12 g of salt per day) and not enough potassium (less than 3.5 g).

High salt consumption and low potassium intake contribute to high blood pressure, which in turn elevates the risk of heart disease and stroke.

Reducing salt intake to the recommended level of less than 5 g per day would avoid 1.7 million deaths each year.

People are usually oblivious of the amount of salt they intake. In many societies, most salt comes from processed foods (e.g. ready meals; processed meats such as bacon, ham, and salami; cheese; and salty snacks) or foods consumed regularly in great amounts(e.g. bread). Salt is also added to foods during cooking (e.g. bouillon, stock cubes, soy sauce, and fish sauce) or at the point of consumption (e.g. table salt).

Salt intake can be reduced by:
limiting the amount of salt and high-sodium condiments (e.g. soy sauce, fish sauce, and bouillon) when cooking and preparing foods
not having salt or high-sodium sauces on the table
limiting the consumption of salty snacks
choosing products with lower sodium content.
Some food companies are reformulating recipes to lessen the salt content of their products, and people should be advised to study nutrition labels to learn how much sodium is in a product before purchasing or consuming it.

Potassium may counterbalance the harmful effects of high salt consumption on blood pressure. Intake of potassium may be increased by consuming fresh fruit and vegetables.

Sugars

In both adults and children, the consumption of free sugars should be lowered to less than 10% of total calorie intake. A reduction to less than 5% of total calorie consumption can provide considerable health improvements.

Consuming free sugars enhances the risk of dental caries (tooth decay). Excess calories from meals and drinks high in free sugars also contribute to unhealthy weight gain, which may lead to overweight and obesity. Recent evidence also demonstrates that free sugars affect blood pressure and serum lipids, and suggests that a reduction in free sugar intake decreases risk factors for cardiovascular disorders.

Sugars intake can be reduced by:

limiting the consumption of foods and drinks containing high amounts of sugars, such as sugary snacks, candies, and sugar-sweetened beverages (i.e. all types of beverages containing free sugars – these include carbonated or non-carbonated soft drinks, fruit or vegetable juices and drinks, liquid and powder concentrates, flavored water, energy, and sports drinks, ready-to-drink tea, ready-to-drink coffee, and flavored milk drinks); and eating fresh fruit and raw vegetables as snacks instead of sugary snacks.

Benefits Of Healthy Diets

Following a balanced diet offers various benefits, including building strong bones, preserving the heart, preventing disease, and enhancing the mood.

Heart health

According to the Centers for Disease Control and Prevention (CDC), heart disease is the main cause of death for persons in the United States.

The American Heart Association (AHA) states that nearly half of U.S. persons live with some sort of cardiovascular disease.

High blood pressure, or hypertension, is an emerging concern in the U.S. The disease may lead to a heart attack, cardiac failure, and a stroke.

It may be possible to avert up to 80% of early heart disease and stroke diagnoses by lifestyle adjustments, such as increased physical activity and healthy nutrition.

The meals people eat may reduce their blood pressure and help preserve their heart's health.

The DASH diet or the Dietary Approaches to Stop Hypertension diet incorporates loads of heart-healthy dishes like:
eating lots of vegetables, fruits, and whole grains
choosing fat-free or reduced fat dairy products, fish, poultry, lentils, nuts, and vegetable oils
minimizing saturated and trans fat consumption, such as rich meats and full-fat dairy products
limiting beverages and meals that include added sugars
reducing sodium intake to fewer than 2,300 milligrams per day — preferably 1,500 mg daily — and boosting consumption of potassium, magnesium, and calcium
High-fiber diets are also crucial for keeping the heart healthy.

The AHA believes that dietary fiber helps improve blood cholesterol and decreases the risk of heart disease, stroke, obesity, and type 2 diabetes.
The medical profession has long recognized the relationship between trans fats and heart-related disorders, such as coronary heart disease.
Limiting certain kinds of fats may also benefit heart health. For instance, reducing trans fats decreases the levels of low-density lipoprotein (LDL)

cholesterol. This form of cholesterol causes plaque to accumulate inside the arteries, increasing the risk of a heart attack and stroke.

Reducing blood pressure may also boost heart health. Most individuals may do this by reducing their salt consumption to no more than 1,500mg per day.

Food makers add salt to many processed and quick meals, and a person who desires to decrease their blood pressure should avoid these goods.

Reduced Cancer Risk

A person may eat foods that contain antioxidants to help reduce their risk of developing cancer by protecting their cells from damage.

The presence of free radicals in the body increases the risk of cancer, but antioxidants help remove them to lower the likelihood of this disease.

Many phytochemicals present in fruits, vegetables, nuts, and legumes work as antioxidants, including beta carotene, lycopene, and vitamins A, C, and E.

According to the National Cancer Institute, there are laboratory and animal studies that relate specific antioxidants to a lower risk of free radical damage linked to cancer. However, human trials are inconclusive and doctors advise against using these dietary supplements without consulting them first.

Foods strong in antioxidants include:

berries, such as blueberries and raspberries

dark, leafy greens

pumpkin with carrots

nuts and seeds

Having obesity may raise a person's chance of acquiring cancer and result in inferior results. Maintaining a modest weight may lessen these hazards.

In a 2014 study, researchers showed that a diet high in fruits lowered the incidence of upper gastrointestinal tract malignancies.

They also discovered that a diet high in vegetables, fruits, and fiber lowers the risk of colorectal cancer, whereas a diet rich in fiber decreases the risk of liver cancer.

Better Mood

Some data reveals a tight association between nutrition and mood.

In 2016, researchers observed that meals with a high glycemic load may provoke higher feelings of sadness and tiredness in persons who have obesity but are otherwise healthy.

A diet with a high glycemic load includes many refined carbohydrates, such as those found in soft drinks, cakes, white bread, and biscuits. Vegetables, whole fruit, and whole grains have a reduced glycemic load.

Recent research also found that diet can affect blood glucose levels, immune activation, and the gut microbiome, which may affect a person's mood. The researchers also discovered that there may be a correlation between more nutritious diets, such as the Mediterranean diet, and greater mental health. Whereas, the reverse is true for diets with large quantities of red meat, processed, and high-fat meals.

It is vital to note that the researchers noted a demand for more study into the processes that connect diet and mental health.

Improved Gut Health

The colon is filled with naturally occurring bacteria, which perform key rolesTrusted Source in metabolism and digestion.

Certain kinds of bacteria also create vitamins K and B, which assist the colon. They may also help fight hazardous germs and viruses.
A diet that is strong in fiber may decreaseTrusted Source inflammation in the stomach. A diet rich in fiber vegetables, fruits, legumes, and whole grains may offer a mix of prebiotics and probiotics that assist healthy bacteria to grow in the colon.
These fermented foods are high in probiotics:
yogurt
kimchi
sauerkraut
miso
kefir
Prebiotics may help relieve several digestive disorders, including irritable bowel syndrome (IBS) symptoms.

Improved Memory
A nutritious diet may assist sustain cognitive and brain function. However, the additional definitive study is essential.
A 2015 research discovered minerals and meals that protect against cognitive decline and dementia. The researchers found the following to be beneficial:
vitamin D, C, and E, omega-3 fatty acids

flavonoids and polyphenols fish
Among other diets, the Mediterranean diet combines several of these components.

Weight Loss

Maintaining a modest weight may help lower the risk of chronic health conditions. A person who has excess weight or obesity may be at risk of having several illnesses, including:
coronary heart disease
type 2 diabetes
osteoarthritis
stroke
hypertension
various mental health problems
some cancers
Many nutritious foods, including vegetables, fruits, and legumes, are fewer calories than most processed meals.
Maintaining a nutritious diet might help a person remain inside their daily limit without tracking their calorie consumption.
In 2018, researchers showed that adopting a diet high in fiber and lean proteins resulted in weight reduction without the necessity for monitoring calorie consumption.

Diabetes Management

A nutritious diet may benefit a person with diabetes:

maintain their blood glucose levels

maintain their blood pressure and cholesterol within goal limits

avoid or postpone the effects of diabetes maintain a modest weight

It is crucial for persons with diabetes to minimize their consumption of meals containing added sugar and salt. They should also consider avoiding fried meals rich in saturated and trans fats.

Strong Bones And Teeth

A diet with appropriate calcium and magnesium is crucial for healthy bones and teeth. Keeping the bones healthy helps lessen the likelihood of bone disorders later in life, such as osteoporosis.

The following foods are high in calcium:

dairy products

kale

broccoli

canned fish with bones

Food makers regularly fortify cereals, tofu, and plant-based milk with calcium.

Magnesium is present in many foods, and some of the finest sources:

leafy green veggies

nuts

seeds

entire grains

Getting Better Sleep

A range of problems, including sleep apnea, may alter sleep patterns.

Sleep apnea happens when a disorder persistently restricts the airways during sleep. Risk factors include obesity and consuming alcohol.

Reducing alcohol and caffeine consumption may help a person get peaceful sleep, whether they have sleep apnea or not.

The health of the future generation

Children acquire most health-related behaviors from the people around them, and parents who model good diet and activity habits are likely to pass them on.

Eating at home may also help. In 2018, researchers discovered that youngsters who regularly ate meals with their family consumed more vegetables and less sugary items than their classmates, who ate at home less often.

Quick Tips For A Healthful Diet

There are many minor methods to enhance a person's diet, including:

swapping soft drinks for water or herbal tea
ensuring each meal consists of some fresh produce
choosing whole grains instead of processed carbs
ingesting entire fruits instead of liquids
reducing red and processed meats, which are rich in salt and may raise the risk of colon cancer
eating more lean protein, which individuals may get in eggs, tofu, fish, and nuts

A person may also benefit from taking a cooking lesson and learning how to integrate more veggies into their meals.

Summary

Healthy eating offers several advantages, such as lowering the risk of heart disease, stroke, obesity, and type 2 diabetes. A person may also increase their mood and acquire more energy by keeping a balanced diet.

Chapter 3

BEST FOOD FOR PREGNANCY

Pregnancy diet

A healthy pregnancy diet should be much the same as your regular healthy diet, just with 340 to 450 more calories per day for the greatest physical and mental health of infants. Food rich in Protein, Carbohydrates, and Iron should be the most significant portion of the diet during this era. Dehydration may lead to a lot of issues and complications in the future, taking a lot of water and other fluids every day keeps you and the baby from difficulty.

An unbalanced diet may create a poor fetus with an immune level, which might cause miscarriage. Now you need to carefully arrange your pregnancy food in a healthy proportion. Excess of anything might produce complications for you and the baby.

As you require a healthy diet for this time, you should avoid and remove certain things from your list notably junk food, alcohol, drinks, and cigarettes

because Nicotine, Alcohol, and Caffeine may really be damaging to the baby and also dehydrates the body. Use only nutritious meals throughout the trimester for a healthy and intellectual baby.
Aim for a healthy variety of foods, including:
complex carbohydrates
protein
vegetables and fruits
grains and legumes
healthful fats
If you currently eat a healthy diet, you'll only need to make modest alterations. Fluids, fiber, and iron-rich meals are particularly vital during pregnancy.

Vitamins and minerals
Pregnant women need bigger quantities of several vitamins and minerals than women who aren't pregnant. Folic acid and zinc are just two examples.

Once you find out you're pregnant, you may wish to increase your vitamin and mineral intake with the help of supplements. Be sure to read nutrition labels and seek your doctor's advice before using any supplements or over-the-counter (OTC) medications.

Although uncommon, consuming supplements might result in vitamin toxicity or overdose. However, a complete prenatal vitamin will generally provide a decent combination of the nutrients that you need for a healthy pregnancy.

Discover the healthy ideal meals during the pregnancy period:

1 Bean: There are types of beans. Black beans, pinto beans, chickpeas. You may select the one that includes fiber and protein. Protein is very important during this period. Beans also deliver Fiber to the body and assist to prevent and treat various ailments. Beans are an excellent source of Iron, Zinc, Calcium, and Foliate.

2. Eggs: Eggs are a major source of protein. Every cell of the infant requires protein. The egg is rich in choline, which stimulates the baby's development and brain function. Besides protein, eggs provide various nutrients in the form of lipids, minerals (such as Zinc and Selenium), and vitamins A, D, and B, which make them an important dietary item during pregnancy.

As eggs are rich in cholesterol hence avoid too many eggs however a healthy individual with normal blood cholesterol may have one to two eggs each day. Avoid using raw eggs since it might generate issues for the digestive system of the mother, which impedes the baby's development.

3. Potatoes and Sweet Potatoes: Potatoes and amp; sweet potatoes provide a significant amount of vitamin A and Iron. This is highly crucial for both the infant and mother.
Vitamin A and Iron are needed for the lining of the eyes, lungs, urinary and digestive systems. It is also needed for lymphocytes or white blood cells that fight against pathogens. Potatoes are highly useful to feed the baby in the womb.

4. Omega-3 (fatty acids): Water fish such as Salmon, Tuna, Sardines, Anchovies and Herring are particularly high suppliers of Omega-3 fatty acids. EPA and DHA are Omega-3 fatty acids that assist the body's heart, brain, eyes, central nervous system, inflammatory response and immunological system.
Adding EPA and DHA to the diet of pregnant women has a good influence on visual and cognitive development of the infant. It is also extremely useful

for the pregnant lady. The daily guideline for the pregnant lady is 300mg DHA and 250mg EPA.

5. Dry Fruits and Nuts: Nuts such as almond, walnut, peanuts are also fantastic sources of Omega-3, calcium and protein which are extremely necessary for the body's brain and development. Almonds are antioxidants against cancer and a very rich source of calcium too.

6. Whole Grains, Oatmeal, and Popcorn: Whole grains are beneficial in pregnancy since they are abundant in fiber and critical minerals like Vitamin E, Selenium, and phytonutrients. As popcorn and oatmeal are complete grains and give general nutrients throughout the pregnancy trimester.

7. Milk and Yogurt: Are rich in protein and a wonderful source of calcium. This calcium is highly important for both the infant and mother. Calcium is a critical vitamin for a baby's bones and teeth. Taking a healthy quantity of calcium is also highly vital for keeping the good health of the skeleton as well.
Daily suggested 1000 to 1300mg, if you do not take enough calcium, start taking calcium to complete the

needs of calcium for the baby's bones and development. The deficiency of calcium may lead to osteoporosis, which can cause loss of bone density.

8. Meats: Meat is a good source of high-quality protein and iron. High protein meal assists in the development of tissues and cells of the baby's body and brain. Use white and fat-free red meat during pregnancy. Eat completely cooked meat and avoid half-cooked and steamed meat since there is a chance of passing on germs and parasites from the meat for you and the baby that may be highly damaging for the infant.

9. Colored Fruits: Eating a diversity of colorful fruits like green, red, orange, yellow, purple, and white fruit helps guarantee that you and the baby are receiving a variety of beneficial nutrients. Apples, Oranges, apricots, Bananas, Grapes, Guavas, Mangoes, Pears, Plums, Peaches, Strawberries, and watermelons are the greatest fruits during pregnancy.

10. Green Leafy Vegetables: During pregnancy green leafy vegetables are the finest source of many critical minerals and vitamins.

Asparagus, Broccoli, Collard greens, Kale, Spinach, and Swiss chard are rich in nutritious minerals and vitamins like A, C, E and K. Iron and Folic acid in green leafy vegetables are particularly vital to delivering blood to the baby to remain healthy in the pregnancy.

Other Best Food Suggestions During These trimesters

First Trimester- 01 to 22 weeks

You will require 250-300 more calories every day in this trimester since, in this first trimester, the baby's most vital organs are the brain's neurological system and spinal cord, heartbeat, eyes, hair, buds, legs, and arms start to grow. In this trimester, increase your meal size and amount carefully, eat six meals instead of three meals daily, and include Omega-3 fatty acids, DHA supplement, folic acid, iron, zinc, vitamin C, and E in your diet.

You may get this in egg yolks, maize oil, walnut, yogurt, citrus fruit, green leafy vegetables, beans, sweet potatoes, salmon, and sardines. You also require additional vitamins for your personal and fetal wellness. For this, you should see your gynecologist for the typical needed amount of any vitamin and supplement before taking it.

Stop smoking and drinking from the first day, it might increase the difficulties for the baby like low weight, hyperactivity, trouble in learning, attention, and speech, or even cause miscarriage. If you consume a healthy diet in the first trimester you make this difficult. Vomiting and morning sickness in the first three months may be remedied by utilizing potassium in your meals regularly. Avoid greasy or fried meals.

Second Trimester- 13-24 weeks

As you start the second trimester the baby requires more energy for speedy development and growth. During this trimester the baby's brain development, muscles, skeletal structural development, and hair follicle growth have begun. So in this trimester, you need high-nutrition meals. Avoid ingesting extra sugar and fats in this trimester, which may contribute to blood sugar in the future.

You should add additional iron, fiber, folic acid, omega-3, and vitamin A, K, B, and E supplements, C (must drink 3-4 glasses of milk daily), and vitamin D to absorb the vitamin C. Food containing these vitamins have a good influence on the baby's weight and height.

You may get fiber in beans, rice, wheat, pasta, and oatmeal. The deficiency of vitamin K may induce serious bleeding. Leafy vegetables and liver are rich sources of vitamin K. For additional vitamins you may include almonds, dates, butter, fish, cheese, yogurt, liver, soybeans, cereals, yeast, milk, groundnut, and fresh vegetables, green veggies, and fruit every day in your suggested diet.

Third Trimester- 25-36 weeks

When you enter the last trimester, some vitamins and minerals are still needed for the good health of the baby and as well the mother's health since in this trimester the main organ (brain, body, and bones), veins, spider veins, skins and development of the kid have been concluded. You need a lot of calories to deliver a healthy baby without difficulties.

You need additional calcium, iron, proteins, folic acid, omega-3 fatty acids, vitamin D, E, and other vitamin supplements. These supplements, vitamins, and minerals (use 8-10 glasses of water every day) may make your delivery smoother.

Taking care of yourself is one of the finest ways to take care of your developing kid.

www.ingramcontent.com/pod-product-compliance
Lightning Source LLC
LaVergne TN
LVHW052104160826
845678LV00015B/3352

* 9 7 9 8 8 4 7 1 3 3 7 1 5 *